Dr. Corrine Morgan
presents

'The
Light
Within You'

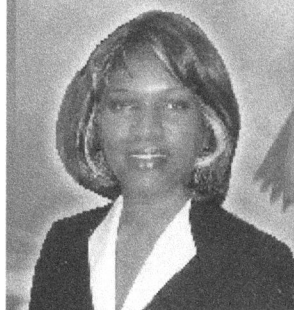

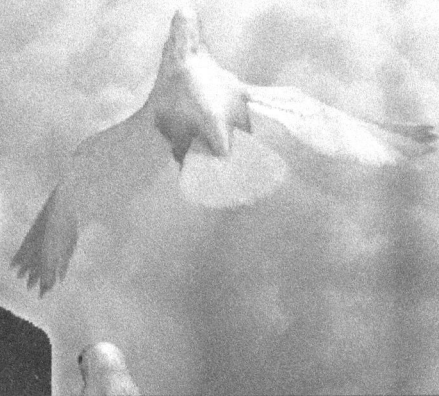

Dr. Corrine Morgan

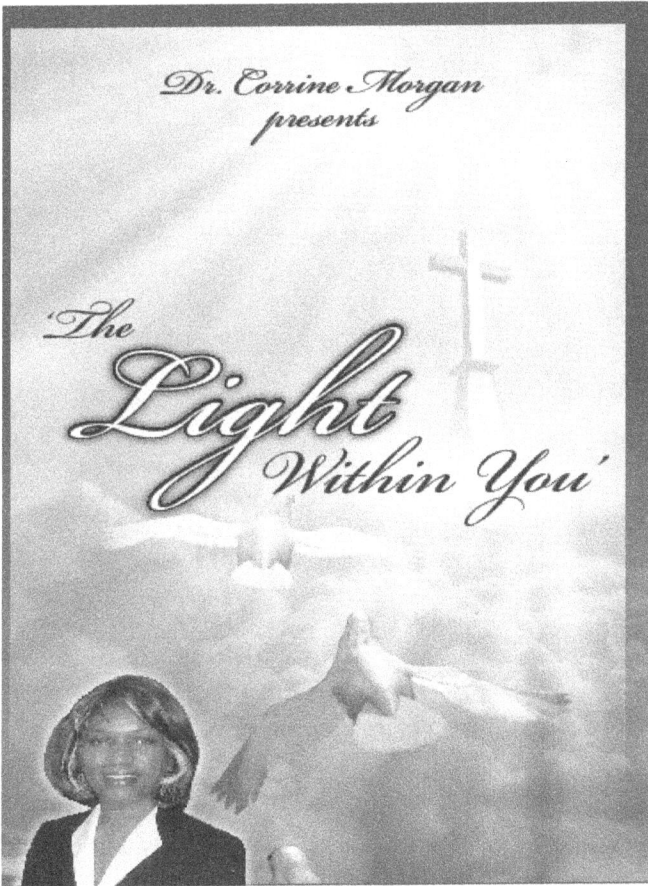

Dr. Corrine Morgan
presents

'The *Light* Within You'

ANOINTED ROSE PRESS™

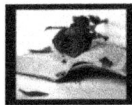

Dr. Corrine Morgan

ANOINTED ROSE PRESS™

The Anointed Rose Press name and logo are registered
Trademarks of ANOINTED ROSE PRESS™

Dr. Corrine Morgan Presents the Light Within You©
Dr. Corrine Morgan
(215) 922-4782
E-mail: drcorrinemorgan@aol.com

ISBN-13:978-0-9826841-6-0
ISBN-10 0-9826841-6-9
© 2011 by Dr. Corrine Morgan

Anointed Rose Press™
P.O. Box 21371
Philadelphia, PA 19141
E-mail: anointedrosepress.@gmail.com

Library of Congress Control Number: 2011902939
Library of Congress Catalog-in-Publication Data

Morgan, Dr. Corrine

Dr. Corrine Morgan Presents the Light Within You / Corrine Morgan
p. cm.
ISBN 0-9826841-6-9 (trade pbk.: alk. paper)

1. Autobiography 2. Spirituality

Cover Design:
THE PRINTED WORD, INC.
Philadelphia, PA (215) 224-5500

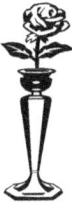

Preface

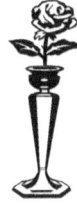

Today, I enjoy life as a doctor of Chiropractic care, a minister, a mentor, a mother and a grandmother. I've been blessed with having accomplished all of this because of a determined spirit and help from many people along the way, and "hearing" the Light within me. The journey has taken me through unexpected trials which have turned into blessings over the years. I have successfully overcome the odds, and broken the cycle of poverty that seemed to loom over my family's future.

The odds were not in my favor, given the circumstances of my early life, growing up in a working class family in the inner city. The cycle of poverty is a condition that many people experience without a clear sense of how to escape. I am a living testimony that you can get here from there.

Early in my life, I was a divorced single mother with three children. Despite outward appearances, I always put God and family first. I never allowed stereotypes to dictate what I could achieve. I learned to view my pitfalls and stumbling blocks as stepping stones. Every step of the way, as I moved toward my goal, 'angels' appeared in my life – people who became friends, mentors, advisors and supporters of my cause. These people galvanized my commitment to serve others. Their assistance to my growth has fostered my dedication to a life of service, particularly in the various neighborhoods where I grew up. Trusting and accepting yourself at every stage helps prepare you for the next level. Education is the key that unlocks lasting opportunities. Surrounding yourself with positive personalities will provide the endorsement you need to succeed.

As a youngster growing up in North Philadelphia, I never expected to become a Doctor of Chiropractic. I never imagined myself standing in front of employees or speaking to large groups of people instructing them on principles of health and wellness. Yet, here I am. And what an amazing journey it has been and continues to be.

My hope is that this book will be an inspiration to people who feel helpless, and enable them to realize they can rise above their circumstances. Remember, there is a light that is part of you; learn how to hold onto the light. If it can happen for me, it can happen for you. My formal statement is, *"I can do all things through Christ who strengthens me."*

Dr. Corrine C. Morgan

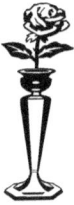

Introduction

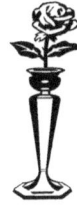

There is a light that is innate in every one of us. I believe this "beam of light" will come out and shine if or when we allow it to. No matter how grim the situation seems to be, we can always call on this light, if we know how to, and let it shine through. Our very essence is very much a part of this light. All we have to do is be silent for a minute and feel that light-force that is within you. Let the Light shine through.

Remember, as you allow this light to come in, God is in control. He is there with you. As we endure all of our troubles, we know we have the light of God.

And His love will always transform us, protect us and be with us; and if we allow it, this light that is God will transform you into the person you are to be. (Wow!)

Dr. Corrine C. Morgan-Rutland

Dr. Corrine Morgan

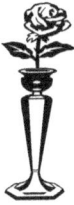

Dedication

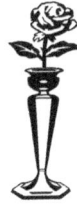

Allen Rutland (*Husband*)

Jeffrey, Jeanine, Joel (*Children*)

Mother Brown (*Mother*)

Brenda (*sister*)

Aunt Evelyn

Grand-Mom Rosie

Grand-Mom Mildred

Smitty (*Friend*)

I dedicate this book with all of my sincere appreciation and gratitude to God, to my family and to all of those who helped me in this lifetime.

Dr. Corrine C. Morgan

Dr. Corrine Morgan

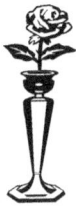

Chapter 1

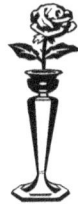

In 1958, a young girl at eight years old was rushed to the hospital with all of her faculties failing. Her heart was racing, and her fever was so high that she had to be put in ice water before the doctors could touch her. Her eyes were rolled up in the back of her head. When they brought her in, the doctors told her mother that, clinically, she was dead, and she would not make it through the night.

They stated that even if there was a glimpse of a chance of her survival, she would be brain dead for the rest of her life. She would never be able to have children because her "private area" had been eaten up with fever. This young girl had gone into a coma. Her mother was told that it was like her brain was an egg and a tomato.

The young girl remembers coming out of her physical body and standing there looking at her lifeless body; just standing there in space like she was waiting for something to happen. She saw herself, but there was nothing humanly possible she could do.

This young girl described her experience at the point of death as seeing a tall man with a dark robe on, pointing at her. She was devastated, however, all she could do was stand there. She remembered every time the man's hand would try to come close to her, there was a bright yellow, very bright light that would stop his hands from touching her. She remembered that the light would burn the man's hand, so he had to remove his hands from her. She remembers this like it happened yesterday; this young woman was me.

Dr. Corrine Morgan

I remember flying into the air, and seeing my mother on her knees crying and saying that she would never drink again. I remember all the members of our Catholic Church praying for me. As they prayed, the light got bigger and brighter.

I remember my grandmother, who was a beautiful small woman of great wisdom, who walked into the room and asked all the doctors to leave. She told my mother to leave, and then my grandmother fell to her knees and prayed, and began to call on the Lord Jesus Christ to heal her granddaughter. As she prayed and cried out to God, the light became brighter and brighter.

I also remember calling my mother's name, telling my mother that I was going to be okay. I remembered when the doctors told my mother that I would not make it through the night, my mother fainted. I was calling my mother, not realizing that my mother could not hear me. They had done all they could do, but the odds seemed impossible. Later that day, my mom went to the funeral parlor to make arrangements.

I remember a tender hand touching me, and someone saying, "You will be alright." The prayer in the light had become so bright that it began to shine all over my body. All of a sudden, my body began to respond. Then, as the nurse counted my death "rattles", I began to come up out of my coma, and said, "Where is my sister?" The nurse got up and ran down the hallway, screaming at the top of her voice, "It's a miracle!"

I remember my hair had burned off from the fever while I was in the hospital. After I came out of my coma, my walking was different and my body felt strange. However, I continued to get well.

In recovery I felt alone, however I knew I was not alone. I always felt someone else is with me, then and now. Personally, I believe all of us have a guardian angel with us to guide and protect us; we must tap into that source. I believe this is here for all of us.

The doctor did all they could do. They worked hard to the best of their capabilities. However, I believe without the touch of the power of God, I would not be alive today. The light shines through.

I know God exists; I experienced Him as I experience Him every day of my life. There is no doubt in my mind that God exists. God exists for all of us. He is a light. The Gospel of John 3:19 talks about the "Light".

Many people don't want their lives exposed to God's light because they are afraid of what will be revealed. They don't want to be changed. Don't be surprised when these same people are threatened by your desire to obey GOD and do what is right; because they are afraid that the light in you may expose some of the darkness in their lives. Rather than giving in to discouragement, pray that they will come to see how much better it is to live in the light than in darkness

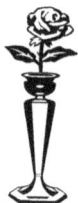

Chapter 2

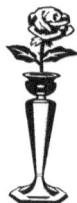

The beginning of my journey in life started when my father died. My mother and father were teenage lovers. They were married at a young age. I could see the love they had for each other when Daddy would come home from work. As I think about this today, I can see a work of art as they would laugh and talk together.

Then, it happened my father who was the life of the family was killed in a car accident. My mother was stunned. All she could do was to stare into space. Then there was the funeral. All the family cried when we saw Daddy. I said to myself, "It cannot be". I think I went into a deep state of depression. I refused to go to school. I stayed by myself. I thought, "How could this happen to me?"

The smile of my Dad was gone. The encouragement to go to college dried up. I would say to myself, what do I do next? My mother started to drink heavily. She would come home at night staggering.

She would leave me and my sister home alone at night. One night I crossed over this wide street in my pajamas and found my mother in a bar. I begged her to come home.

One night I remember one of her friends fondled me. After I started to cry, he left me alone. I tried to tell Mom but she would not hear it. My cousin came over one night and raped me, then ran away laughing. It is strange, but shortly after that he died of some disease. I remember looking in his coffin and telling him how I forgave him for what he had done to me.

I never told anyone until later when I went to treatment.

When I say I forgave him for what he had done to me, it was later. I had taken one of my mentees for counseling due to her being molested as a child. This is when I forgave my cousin for what he had done to me. I remember the counselor talking to her and I began to rock back and forth and started sweating. Then I got up and ran out of the room. The counselor came out and began to talk to me. It was wild; I realized that I needed counseling and did receive it.

As I talked to someone about my situation, the light was there with me. I also learned that so many of us have hidden issues and we must let them go. This is one of many ways that our light can and will shine through. I have also learned that all of us have lights that are around us at all times. The lights are there to protect us. As we let go and let God, our light will shine.

Growing up, the house we lived in was in the worst section. My mother finally got up enough courage to move on her own. We lived in a rat and roach infested place. It was terrible. We did the best we could do. I could only guess that was all that she could afford. One night I got bitten by a rat and there were marks on my body. The State came to take away my sister and myself from our mother because of what the neighbors saw. My mother put us in Catholic school. During that time, I asked the Lord to come into my heart, and He did.

Then it happened that I got very sick and was rushed to the hospital profusely sweating. I went into a coma, and I was told my eyes went up into the back of my head. My head felt like it was going to explode any minute. My body was riddled with sores and bites from the rodents in the apartment. 911 was called.

I remember waking up in the hospital and all these people around me trying to help me, putting me in ice so my fever would come down. I was also seeing a little light there. At this young age, I asked the Lord to come into my life and He did. What a light that was!

This was the time when I came out of my body, seeing my family praying for me, and seeing a man with a grey long suit pointing his finger toward me. All I could do was to stand there next to my body. It seems like it was yesterday when my spirit was wandering around the church watching people praying for me and seeing my mother stating, "Please help my child." I was standing next to her but she could not see or hear me. I have learned from that experience that there are spirits who watch us, and care. This was my own experience; it was real and it happened to me.

While in the hospital, the doctors told my mother if I would live I would be a vegetable all of my life, and that all of my life they would have to put me into a home. They said I would never have children because my insides were torn up, and all I had to look forward to was a life in an institution.

However, the strong bright light inside of me proved all of them wrong. Let me assure you the doctors did all they could, but we serve a mighty God that can do all things.

After I had the incident in the hospital, my mother changed. I believe it was a wake-up call for Mom and the family. Once I came out of the hospital, my mother stopped drinking and she got a job at Campbell Soup Company. She learned the trade of cooking at Campbell Soup.

She became the top chef and worked there for many years. It is funny how I never could cook, only boil water (smile).

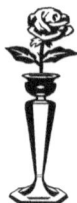

Chapter 3

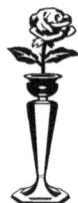

As for myself, I went back to school, once I was home. After the experience in the hospital, I continued to feel alone even though I knew someone was there with me.

Time began to pass and I began to get healthier. With all of the chaos around me, I managed to continue to go to school. I remembered my father would say,

"When you go to college." So, I went from a high school to a business school, not realizing what I had done. I graduated business school at 16 with a 3.8 point average. At that time all my friends were getting married and I thought it was the best thing to do.

I tried with all my heart and soul to do the right thing. I remember feeling alone; and then I met this man. I had my eyes on this tall manly beautiful man who looked like my father. We got married and had a fairly big wedding. We were supposed to live happily ever after, so I thought. We just knew that getting married was the right thing to do. The problem was God was there but not on board with us.

After the divorce, my life was in chaos. At first, I went from man to man to man, and then I realized I was not my mother. The problem was because of my belief, I was too scared to have sex with them; and I was constantly afraid that someone would try to molest my children the way I had been. I was made to feel dirty about myself. I felt so ashamed;

I felt like I was the worst person on earth. My marriage to this man had failed. No one wanted to be around me. I was in a state of limbo. We went to court, and he was supposed to pay for child support, but he moved out of state. I could not find him; he seemed to have disappeared – no man, no support – what to do?

When we were together, I worked in the customer service department at Blue Cross/Blue Shield. He watched the children at night and I stayed at home during the day.

One day I was desperate; I had to find a job because the funds were gone. I didn't know what to do. I went to Blue Cross to see if I could work part-time. In the meantime I heard that Mr. Ex. had moved to Patricia Drive in Yeadon, PA. Still, I don't know how I found out about that.

Anyway, as I was waiting for a job application downtown, there was this elderly lady having a hard time with her insurance. I remembered I had worked the office before, therefore I knew insurance. I asked her could I help her, and she said "yes". I looked at her policy and told her exactly what her policy meant!! The older lady was elated. She thanked me over and over. It just so happened that I looked at her address, and it looked like where I heard that Mr. Ex. was. Could it be?

I described him to her and told her he was an old friend. She told me exactly where he and his "wife" lived (I was the real wife). This man owed me over $4,500 for child support and arrears. This could only be God. I went home that afternoon and cried. The next day I went directly to the apartment building and I saw his car.

My heart fell to the floor. The outside door of the building was locked, and I had to find a way in. As I walked around the apartment building trying to find a way to get in, I saw an open window leading to the second floor. I was not going to leave without something. I had already told the girl across the street who was watching my children, if I was not back that night to call my family or #911.

I stood on top of a red car and jumped into the window. I was in, and all I had to do was to find him. As I looked down on the bell-board for his address, my heart leaped out when I saw his name as Mr. and Mrs. I could have fainted but I did not. As I walked up the steps to the upper apartment, my heart began to beat louder and louder. By the time I knocked on the door, I could hardly breathe.

As I knocked on the door, I asked God to be with me. I needed that light since I did not know if I would be killed or beaten up or what. So, when he opened the door, the Lord said to say nothing, and I didn't. I just put my hand out for the check and he handed it to me. It is strange that as I left that apartment building, I did not look back, and I have never looked back since that date.

I knew I had to do something in my life, but what to do? I always wanted to be a doctor, but that was "Mission Impossible" because I felt so bad about myself – lower than a snake. However, I could not stay there and so something had to give. There was something missing in my life.

One day as I felt terrible about myself and having a self pity party, I saw a man on television with beautiful white hair. This man's message was, "You can be the person you want to be". He stated, "All you have to do is apply yourself." He also stated, "All you have to do is put God first; have faith in God and have faith in yourself." And he said, "Don't worry about it, just do it."

At that moment I saw the light. I was ready but I did not know where to go, so I had to wait on the Lord. This has stayed with me throughout my life time. And I want to thank you Dr. Robert Schuller.

Can you imagine how I felt when I later met Dr. Schuller and was introduced as "Dr. Corrine Morgan?" Thank God for the light. I had to pinch myself because this was a dream that came through.

Matthew chapter 5 teaches us we are the light of the world. A city that is set on a hill cannot be hidden. Nor do they light a lamp then put it under a basket, but on a lamp stand, and it gives light to all who are in the house. Let your light so shine before men, that they may see your good works and glorify your Father in heaven. As we live for Christ, we will glow like the light that shines through us

Then, my good friend Millie told me about a class at the local church. I started going to the class, which I breezed through. My girlfriend was surprised, but not as surprised as I was. I could not believe this. I actually took a class and passed it. I said to myself, "I am not as stupid as I think I am." I took another class and passed it.

This gave me a new lease on life. I said to myself, that I knew I had to change my lifestyle. I found myself a new breed of people who were positive and upbeat, and who wanted to do something with their lives. I left all my negative friends alone, who would "prey" on others instead of "praying" for them.

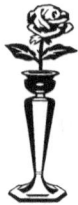

Chapter 4

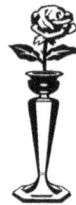

I was divorced and on welfare by the age of 24, with 3 children. I was alone, scared and had nowhere to go. I began working at night, cleaning toilets, cleaning people's houses, cleaning buses or doing whatever work I could find.

Again, I was alone, but I did not feel alone. There was something there; an existence I did not know how to tap into

until later. I felt ugly and unwanted.
How could this happen to me? I did not
know which way to turn. My life was in
chaos. I could only turn to the Lord for
my life.

I remember falling down on
my knees crying and asking God
Almighty to help me. I felt so alone, except
for the presence of God. I felt abandoned
by my family except for my grandmother.
However, that strange little light was ever
present. My friends and everyone was
gone; there was only God to be with me.

One day my aunt Evelyn came over, and all the family was talking about my state of depression after the marriage break-up. However, Aunt Evelyn was the only one to openly talk about it to me, and I did not hear her.

Aunt Evelyn made me get on my knees and pray. She made me stay there until I could feel a difference in my attitude. I was there on my knees, and it seemed like all night and the next day. I felt something happening. I could not figure out what, but it was there – something different.

I remember I was in debt with all the bills. I had to get on welfare. I felt bad about this, however I felt there was no way out; I could not borrow money.

I remember I walked outside my door and asked a strange man to borrow $ 10 dollars because I was broke. I hated to, but I had to go on welfare. At that time I had to turn my house over to the state to get a check. It was very humiliating too, but what to do?

I received a check for $500 a month and we had to live off that money to do the best we could do. The bills kept mounting and all of the money was going for bills. I found myself going into a state of depression but for some reason the light stayed with me. At one time I felt there was no way out: why am I here? What good am I? But a spirit inside of me kept me going. I knew there had to be a better way and I was going to find it. The light would follow me around.

One day I went to my grandmother's house and told her what happened. That day she gave me $ 40. She said $20 is for you and $20 is for those children. She said, "Put God first and make this money grow."

Later, I went to a handbag demonstration, and there was a woman who sold beautiful lady's handbags for a living. Something inside said that I could do this. I took my $20 from my grandmother and whatever other money I had and made a purse for my mother for her birthday. The girls at her job loved it. Then I made some more little bags from the scraps I had at home. To my surprise, women paid me for my handbags. Later, I met a gentleman who knew where to buy bags from in New York, and he showed me how to sell the handbags. I began to sell these bags and made enough money to pay my bills.

That light was shining inside of me. I would say to myself, "Shine light, shine." (smile) There I learned ,,,With God all things are possible... WOW!

With my good friend Millie I continued to go to school at the church learning things that I did not realize I did not know. Now it was time to move ahead. In my head, I heard voices, saying "go back to school." I felt I could do it, but I have these children. What do I do? Where do I start? I continued going to classes at

church, but then it was time to move on.
By the grace of God, I started attending
Community College. However, I did not
realize I had graduated from a non-
accredited high school.

I had to meet with the assistant
dean, she looked at me in my face and
said people like me would never make
anything out of their lives. She said, "You
just do not have it, and will probably
collect a check for the rest of your life."
Was she wrong? That night I went home
and cried and I slapped myself on the face
and said this would never happen again. I

looked up and that light was looking at me. I knew what I had to do.

The next day I went to the dean's office. I wanted to talk to the "big cheese", the dean of students. At first he didn't have any time to talk to me. I threw myself in front of him and all the students, and then he invited me to his office. He looked up my records and found out I did need a High School diploma, and he told me about the GED program. I learned all about the GED. Once I learned that I had to do this, I studied with all of my heart and soul.

Later, I began to teach the GED to "women of the night". We all learned from one another. Seeing Asst. Dean later at Textiles, God showed me humility through all of my experiences. As I taught these women how to read and write, they taught me the meaning of life – what to do and what not to do. (Never judge a book by its cover). God is always with me in everything that I do – Everything, I say!

I continued and by the grace of God I got into Community College. College was rough, but I made it through. The children were in bed by 6 p.m. every night; they hated it. However, we had to do this.

Community College gave me the courage to stay in school. It helped me to realize how important education is.

In undergrad, especially at Community College, it was great because I was home and I had someone to watch my children. My family was my life. At that time I knew I had someone at my grandmother's house to help, however when I started graduate school later, it was a different world. You really had to know your stuff. There wasn't time for any games.

Again, in undergrad school I had to learn how to stop talking ghetto and start talking English. It was like learning a foreign language. I had to remember, "We fall down; but we get up." (smiles) The Thanksgiving and Christmas holidays were very difficult. I only had enough money to feed the children. I remember my mother came over and she would give us the scraps from the residents that lived at the nursing home. It was hard times but I continued going to school, and I continued to make the best out of each situation. I never told anyone about this.

Later, after graduating from Community College and realizing what my dreams were, I wanted so much to be a doctor. While in school, there were so many opportunities, and I found a 5 year program that one of the medical schools had. It was a way to get into medical college, and I jumped on it.

I was scared, but I figured if others could do it, I could do it too. To my surprise, I got in. When I received the letter of acceptance, I fell on my knees and thanked the Lord, "Lord, we did it." I remember sitting in medical school with all the big shots, and sweating bricks because at last I was there.

During that time, my mother had severe back pain, where she was bent over and could only look up at me. She would watch the children for me while I was in school. I remember her complaining of the severe pain that she had every day.

Our family took her to different medical doctors; the doctors did all they could do. They gave her plenty of medicines, however the pain was constant. The Doctors helped but the pain was always present.

All we could do was wish mom the best, we knew she would not be operated on. She did not want to have an operation.

Later, my mother went to a special Doctor, this doctor made her stand taller and helped her to stop her pain I saw a personality change in her. She was happier than before; she was going back to being "Mom". That special doctor was a doctor of Chiropractic.

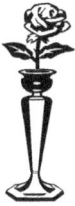

Chapter 5

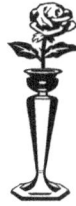

When I realized my Mom was going to see a chiropractor, I immediately looked into the possibilities that chiropractics had to offer. All I could see was the happiness that my mother had, the pain that was not there anymore, the energy she had, and the smiles on her face. I was sold. It was wonderful. One day while in Medical School I looked up and immediately quit school and started chiropractic school. All my friends thought I was crazy, however, they didn't see what I saw in my Mom.

When I decided to go to chiropractic school, I was ridiculed by the family doctors; and people who I thought were my friends told me I would never make anything out of my life. They would say, "You must be crazy." However, the light was with me the whole time. Although it has been over twenty-five years, it seems like it was yesterday. I decided I would pack up my children and head for Iowa, never to come back unless I had "doctor" on the back of my name.

Before I left Philly to go to Iowa, my aunt Evelyn prayed for me in front of everybody. She said, "God take care of this fool, guide her and protect her. Bring her back safe and sound". The Lord led me and my children there in peace with no problem.

I drove to the school. I had a "Hoop-dee" car. If the car started, "Hoop-dee!". If the car stopped, "Hoop-dee!" I asked God to be with me, and He was. I drove from Philadelphia to Iowa in about 2 days. I was on a mission, and God was with me, and I felt the light. Halleluiah!

I remember when I arrived in Iowa in the middle of the night; I went to the place where I was supposed to stay. When they saw that I was African-American, their cold hearts turned me and my children away. I did not have any place to go, as I drove through the city trying to find a place to stay.

As I stood outside of the place where we were supposed to stay, a little man walked up to me and told me about a hotel in this city that had a room for me and the kids. It is strange when I think about it now that this little man looked like the man that I had to borrow the ten dollars from previously. It couldn't be, or could it? Was he one of my angels? Who knows?

I did find the hotel and stayed there. It was a hotel inn down the street, where only the "women of the night" and "Joes" stayed. I knew how to handle the situation because I had previously learned about them from the women that I taught in the GED program. These women in Iowa watched my children for one week until I found a place to stay. The light was shining again - what else could it be??

When I got to the school, I knew I was in the right place. There was only one African American woman before me at the school, but I did not care. All I wanted to do was learn. When I walked in the school, the admissions officer said, "We have a double minority here." When he looked at me, I said, "Who???"

At first, school was very difficult. I had to make sure my children were okay. By then they were in school also. They nicknamed me "The lady in the shoe." When the dean would see me with the kids, he would shake his head and keep moving.

They had no idea what I was doing. I was selling lady's handbags at night. There were no welfare checks for me so I had to do something to take care of my family. It was hard work. However I was on a mission. That "Light" was with me. In graduate school, dealing with parenthood and the demands of the graduate curriculum, the pressure was severe. The existence of God kept me through those hard times.

The fact that the school I attended was predominantly male, with just a few women; and being an African American did not make things any better.

However, God's presence was always there. The teachers, and the students alike, would wonder if I was going to last another day because the drop-out rate in the school was sky high. I realized that the power of the light in me was there to keep me.

I know that God's existence led me to "Smitty" the clean-up lady. She was there talking to me when I needed someone to talk to. I had a boyfriend in Philadelphia who would constantly call me. At first the situation at school was devastating. I went to Smithy and she said, "You must finish school. Once you finish School you decide whatever you want to do. You're here to finish school aren't you?"

"Yes, ma'am!" I loved Smitty. She may have been a cleaning woman, but she was my pillar of strength. When I talked to her I would see that light shine through. Every day I would thank God for her. Unfortunately, not everybody saw Smitty that way. You know every class has a class clown. Well, there was this one guy in our class named Harry. He saw me talking to Smitty one day. In front of the whole class, he said, "Hey Corrine, is that your Mammy?" Just like that.

I looked at him and all this temper came up in me. I said to him, "No, she's not my mother, but because she is - I am. Because she's cleaned these walls in this school, I can sit next to you. Because of all her struggles in life, she has paved the way for me and other people like me to go to school and become a doctor." I was really emotional about it. I told them, "She is my pillar of strength. Because of her I can pave the way for others to come after me." Harry and his friends backed off.

No one bothered me after that. I know God put Smitty in my life. She was a mother to me when I needed a mother to talk to. She was a friend because she realized how lonely I was, trying to make it in a predominately white world. She would give me advice only a woman of color could give to another woman of color. She made sure I could go to church with my family. Only the Lord could send me such a wonderful person.

One time I wanted to quit. I was tired of selling the handbags at night. I was a walking zombie. I told Smitty, "I cannot take it anymore. She said to me, "They let you in, didn't they?" I said, "Yes." "Then keep on," she said.

My other friends encouraged me also, they said, "Always remember who you are and keep on keeping on." I would think, "Remember that light is with me."

Then I found out how wrong I could be about other people. My friends who were White would help me with the children and with my studies. I learned that when you put forth an effort to do the best you can do, there are good friends no matter what color or gender that will help you. I had never realized how much God is a part of us, how we are the same but yet different, and how we all have challenges. There are different strokes for different folks, and if we all learn these lessons, what a great place we could live in. There is nothing that is impossible with God. If I can do this, than you can too.

The light would show with my positive friends, like my friends Dr. Shaw, Dr. Kathy, and Dr. Lory, just to name a few. We were all in this together.

Light has shown again when I met my present husband, who is a wonderful man and has been a role model for my children. Light shows through the friends I have today which are my true friends.

There are also other amazing things that have happened to me. Against all odds, I became the first African American female to be licensed in the State of Pennsylvania. Against all odds, I was featured in Essence magazine and been given the opportunity to travel the world . I have realized that in life we are all part of each other.

Three years after arriving in Davenport, I graduated from Palmer College. I took my first job in Iowa with Dr. Strang. He always said that people are different and that they need to be adjusted differently; depending on where they live.

He told me, "You know the inner city, but you also need to learn about ways of life." He suggested that I move around the country a little before settling down. So that's what I did. I did what my mentor told me to do.

I took an associate position in Arizona. It was beautiful there. It was like paradise. I stayed in Arizona for a year. Then I got a job offer in Louisiana that I could not refuse. They offered to pay me twice as much as the job in Arizona. It was a trip working in Louisiana. The people called me "Yankee."

I went back to Philadelphia to visit my grandmother. She said to me, "Coco, It's time for you to come back to Philadelphia."

"Why?" I asked her. She said, "look! I'm going to die. Your mother's not well. And when I die, someone needs to take care of her or she's gonna die too." I always listened to my grandmother, so in 1988, I packed up the kids and moved back to Philly.

The truth is part of me always wanted to come back. I knew how underserved my community was. They

were being pressured to take all this
medication when they didn't have to. I
knew I had to make a difference. When I
came back to the city, I realized that it was
different. Seeing my people and others
who were really sick, I realized again there
are no mistakes in the universe.

Let that light shine through. Face up
to your problems no matter how bad they
are. Remember, you can choose to
determine your destiny. Remember that
even in the midst of turmoil, the light
(God) is in control. No matter how bad
your situation is, there is always someone
who is worse off. Give support to those who

need it by loving them, and help their light shine through. Challenge someone to join you in showing their light to you. Encourage those who are timid that the light is in God's promises.

With all that I have gone through to get to where I am, I want to let you know you too, can rise above whatever circumstances you encounter. I came from the ghetto, and what I realize is, it's only a state of mind. I came back to the community to serve the very community that fostered my growth.

Everything starts with you – it's always an inside job. As long as you are living, you have the ability to make powerful changes in your life. You must first realize, "I can do this," and once you embrace that fully, you can let the light shine through.

There are many people that we admire for their success who come out of similar and worse situations than you may be experiencing now. T. D. Jakes, Dr. Robert Schuller. Joel Olsten, and the late Reverend Leon Sullivan are just a few. Sometimes disappointment, tragedy and hardship can be the very impetus for your turnaround.

Through it all, you must keep the faith. Someone once said, that "No man or women is an island." The wonderful thing about people in your life, wanted and unwanted, is that they represent a leavening and assurance that your sadness will not be with you always.

We are just an attitude away from the success we've only dreamed of. However, we are all blessed to be a blessing to others. I have been the recipient of unmerited favor many times. People have come into my life that have embraced my spirit and desire to achieve that which God has placed on my heart to share. Their endorsement and support has helped me to realize my goals of becoming, not just a professional, but a person that is essentially a servant to others.

It has been an amazing journey; one that continues to amaze me every day. My early life was a rocky road filled with disappointment enough that could snuff out any hope for success? But I am here to tell you that God is able, and He has been with me through it all. I am here to tell you, if I can do this, you can too. When you think positive and put God first in your life, positive forces will bring positive results to you.

First of all - to change your conditions, start thinking differently, realizing the power is within you. Realign yourself, then do it. You have power to tap into that light. There is a champion within you, just let it out and let it shine. The light within you will serve you.

You must believe and state to yourself, "With God, all things are possible;" then do it. God has a plan for you just like He has a plan for me.

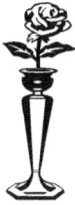

Chapter 6

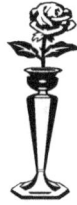

I learned in school the importance of health is critical. I've learned how important it is to care for our bodies – spiritually, mentally, nutritionally, physically and all around. Later, as I began to treat my patients, I saw a need for spiritual help.

Today, I came into the hairdresser's to get my hair done. To my surprise, another girl was there also – even before she knew who I was, we were in prayer. Her husband just died, her favorite brother also died and she was on all kinds of medicine. She was a mess, and she cried and cried and cried.

Before I knew it, we were in deep prayer, giving everything to Jesus, asking Him to hold her up, rebuking the devil in the name of Jesus. Right in front of my eyes, I saw her change. I saw a sparkle of light come into her face; Jesus had her, and that was all that she needed.

In life we need to know that there is a light that shine within all of us. When you truly believe you can - you can. There is a miracle in each one of us. With your belief and trust and the courage to do it - let's do it. Follow your dreams; they are a part of you.

I believe the main secret to life is thanking God for the light that belongs to you. Carry that light with you wherever you go. Never be afraid, you are not alone. Never forget what makes you happy, and laugh. Think on the small items that make you happy.

Dr. Corrine Morgan

Use the time you have here on earth to be the best you are. Always go for the best you can be. Be yourself and enjoy every moment you have with yourself.

Give your worries to God; He has a big shoulder, He made us and He knows what to do.

Whatever dreams you have, let that light shine on them and follow through. I believe faith, trust, and belief are all you need to make it today. Each day take it as a challenge. Take the challenge and let the light shine through you as it continues to shine through me.

We all ministers in our own way and God knows where your heart is. Every day that you wake up, it is a miracle. All of the systems in our body work in synch. Nothing is out of proportion. Walking, talking and doing whatever everyone does naturally. Every day is a miracle. The existence of God is so evident in everything we do. I have learned through the years just to trust in Him, and everything will be alright.

The Lord called me to become one of His ministers. It was October 17, 2009 when I was being ordained as Bishop, that I was saying to myself, "What am I doing here?" I was scared because I did not want to offend God. As I got on my knees, I felt the presence of all my ancestors. I felt my two grandmothers and my great grandmother. I felt my mother and my great aunts and uncles. When I looked at the Bishop who was ordaining me, his voice resonated to me, "You will be the Bishop of Health, and you will heal."

I realize that healing is in us, who we are, how we eat and how we treat our wonderful bodies, as well as how you care for yourself and others.

I realize that the power within us is greater than we can imagine.

You can be the person you want to be. You can show love, turn on the light and let it shine through you.

I believe my life is just beginning. The light is there for all of us to tap into. Use your blessings and this is for you, and you, and especially you.

Dr. Corrine Morgan

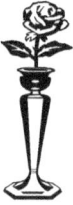

About the Author

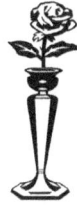

ARTICLE (Reprinted from 2004)

Dr. Corrine Morgan: Believing broke down the barriers

Many people overcome obstacles to go to Chiropractic College; some sacrifice high-paying jobs to follow their passions. Some depend on spouses to support the family until they earn their degree. Many – perhaps most – take out big student loans for financial support.

But few people have had the experiences of Corrine Morgan: She overcame the barriers of racial discrimination, single-parenthood and dire poverty to achieve her coveted goal – a doctorate of chiropractic from Palmer College.

Dr. Morgan earned that degree in 1988. Today she runs a thriving chiropractic practice in South Philadelphia, her hometown. And perhaps, more important – she has mentored dozens of young women to help them overcome their own personal barriers and achieve their dream of becoming a doctor.

Her selflessness has been recognized: She has been nominated for a variety of awards, including Woman of the Year, Chiropractor of the Year and Alumni of the Year. She has also been featured in

Essence Magazine as a role model for other young black women. Dr. Morgan's story is an inspiration to anyone who wonders whether she has what it takes to succeed.

She left her mother's home at 16, lived with her grandmother for a year and married at 17. At 22, she was divorced with three preschool children, no real education and no job.

Racial discrimination – from being denied jobs because of her color to having to fight for an opportunity to get an education – has been no stranger to Morgan.

Many students go to school on a shoestring; Dr. Morgan did it on less than that. To pay the rent, she sold pocketbooks from door-to-door in the evenings. Later, she found low-income housing for $19 month, where she lived until she finished her degree.

Dr. Morgan now practices with her son, who has followed in his mother's footsteps. Part of what she loves is passing on what she has learned to others, especially to young women from all over the country – Arizona, Louisiana, Iowa, South Carolina, Texas, Oregon, and Alaska. They all ask her for advice.

She tells them: *"If I could do this, you can do this. But you have to have faith and focus on what you want. If you apply yourself, there's no reason you can't succeed."*

www.ingramcontent.com/pod-product-compliance
Lightning Source LLC
LaVergne TN
LVHW091205080426
835509LV00006B/839